From Sleep Deprivation To Sleep Tight

With 12 Effective Yoga Poses

By Suchi Gupta

# From Sleep Deprivation To Sleep Tight With 12 Effective Yoga Poses

Dedicated to YOU!

May you achieve your goal of "Good night's sleep"
very soon!

That's my wish for you!

# Table Of Contents

## Acknowledgements

I wish to thank my husband Saket for always showing confidence in me, even when I was not sure of myself! That matters a lot to me.

A big thank you to my families for giving me time and support always. It really helped me while I was busy creating this book.

A very special thanks to Dr. Ken Evoy and everyone at Site Build It! for sharing their expertise and giving advice and guidance on creating this book.

I am truly thankful to the universe every day for all the wonderful people, things and events in my life.

I wish you all the very best on your journey from no sleep / can't sleep to sleep tight / sleep better!!

Natural Sleep Aids to Good Night's Sleep at **Home Without Spending a Penny**!

Plus get to know what are the best **direction** and the best **position** to sleep in!

And 4 **Acupressure** points for sound sleep plus 3 simple **breathing** techniques to take care of your 'can't sleep' woes!!

Along with 40 sleep **tips** and 15 **stress buster** ideas

Plus simple and easy ideas for before-bed **snacking**!!!

# Introduction

Do you always feel tired, sleepy, restless or easily irritable because of lack of sleep? ...or you are using sleeping pills?

Or you are desperate to fall asleep but when you touch the bed, sleep just vanishes?

Would you like to really sleep well, sleep fast...like

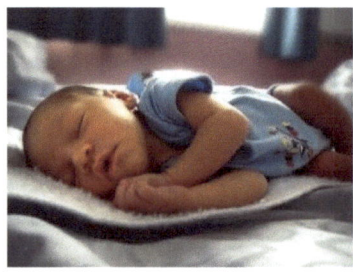 ...a baby...and feel fresh and energetic when u wake up, ready to really live your life your way?

If your answer is Yes, then this book is for you.

Here is what I have for you in this book...

...Some **simple, easy-to-follow and most relaxing** Yoga poses and natural sleep aids to help you to sleep.

You can easily apply these in your daily life, from comfort of your home, without disturbing your schedule.

These postures and tips to sleep tight are simple and **anyone can do them**.

Plus I have **pictures** that clearly show what is to be done. That will also make for an interesting read.

So, no need to spend your hard earned money

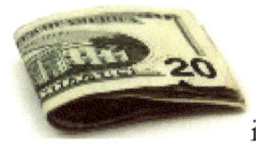

in sleeping pills or visiting doctors.

No need to set aside

...time for appointment with a doctor...No more sleepless nights!

...and I include 15 simple **Stress buster** ideas, just in case you feel stress is the reason you have disturbed or no sleep!

...and I also share with you 4 **acupressure** points that will help you sleep!

...and would you like to know simple **breathing** techniques to sleep better?

And I have included here 40 proven sleep **tips** that are completely natural, no over-the-counter-sleep-aids at all!

Apart from  ideas for yummy bed time **snacking**!

So you can say Goodnight to insomnia and **sleep your way to better health, better body, bigger success and better life!!!**

## How to get the most out of this book

---Implement the poses and tips when you go through this book. Do not just read the book and see the pictures. **Take action and apply** these practical tips for restoring healthy sleep! That will produce results!

---Give yourself time! It may take a few days before these poses/tips/exercises show effect. Have

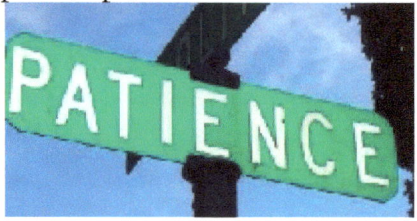

---Keep this 'when you can't sleep at night' book handy so that you can go back to it if you need to.

---Try and see which of the solutions I have shared work for you. You do not need to do them all. Just see **what works best for you**.

# Before you start, Take care!

---I'm not a sleep specialist, these are my **personal experiences** - What works for me and for most people! If you are on a sleep medicine, please understand that the exercises and tips do not replace your medicine.

You may gradually feel like you are able to sleep even without medicine. But make sure you consult your doctor before taking any such step.

---Everybody's body, lifestyle, habits, situations are different. So, observe **what helps you sleep best** and add that to your schedule so that it becomes your habit. You don't need to do all of it.

**---** Doing these exercises **consistently** ONLY will give any results. It's like 'sleep training'.

---Try finding the **root cause** for not being able to sleep.

If its stress or you have a medical condition, what I share in this book may help a bit but not much in the long run. So, solve the root cause first. You may try the **stress management /reduction tricks** that I have shared here, that I use.

...Ok, that's enough word of caution. So, are you ready for what-to-do-when-you-can't-sleep?

Great! Lets' start with a very important sleep well tip...

## The Best Sleep Direction

...is with the **head towards east** with feet pointing towards the west.

Let me make it a little clearer...It means when you lie down your head is in the direction from where sun rises.

Can't have the bed arranged so that you sleep with your head towards east?

No problem!

The second best direction is with the head towards the west, the third choice is south.

But NEVER sleep with your head towards

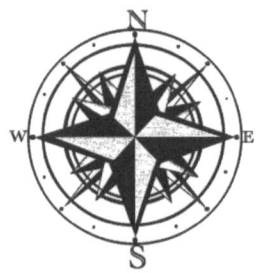

...North. You will experience sleepless nights.

Why?

Let me explain the scientific logic...

Did you know our bodies have a **magnetic field** just like earth?

Yes!  Our head is the north side and feet are the south.

So, if we place our head in north position, the north side of the earth will repel us. Same poles repel!

This can cause disturbed sleep, sleeplessness, headache or heaviness and disturbed blood circulation. It also hinders with the process of digestion.

My mom is always very particular of this and I could never understand why until I read the scientific reason behind it.

That's one very important fact among the sleep facts! Sleep right!!!

Time for a little 'sleep naturally' **nugget**...

One must not have his feet pointing directly towards a door while lying down. That position is called 'Coffin Position' and you know from the word what that would mean.

Ok, now would you like to know the...

## Best Position to Sleep

Just lie down on the bed on your left side so that right leg is over the left leg.

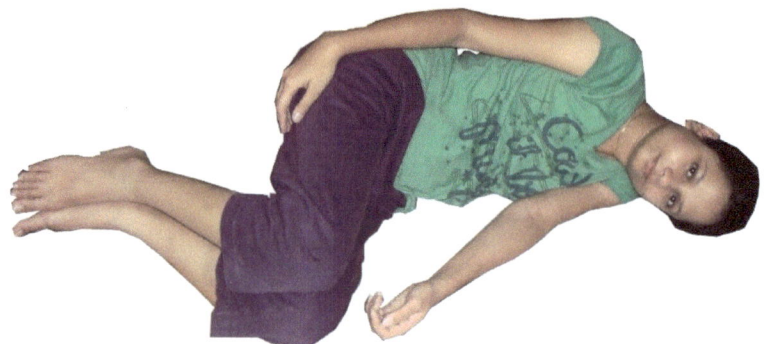

One of the reasons why this is the best among all sleep positions? ...because the blood flows towards the heart. That's why it is the best way to sleep.

I feel so relaxed when I lie down like that. Feels great! Try it!

So simple isn't it? :)

But, you can change it after some time or should I say we tend to change it, which is fine. It's not advisable to keep a constant posture all night.

Now let's go for some of the...

# Best Yoga Poses For Sleep

When to do them? ...**just before you sleep**.

Just a little word of caution...Do them in **moderation to start** with and then you can repeat them more number of times.

So, here we go with one of the **easiest** sleep yoga pose...

# Corpse Pose

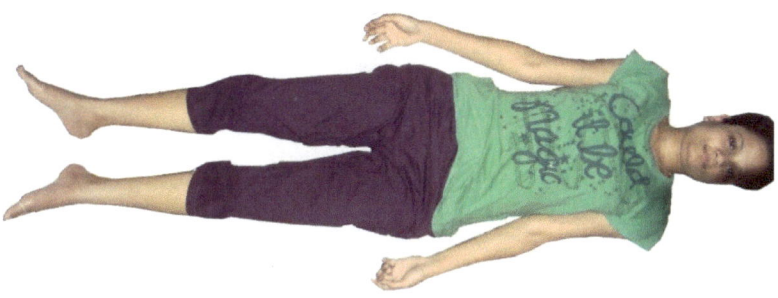

## How to do:

---Just lie down on your bed.

---Keep your hands and legs straight and relax.

This posture is called "Shav-aasana" where "Shav" means corpse.

This is one of the most relaxing poses! Try it! I'm sure you will feel completely relaxed.

I used to do unknowingly since childhood!

# Sitting twist Pose

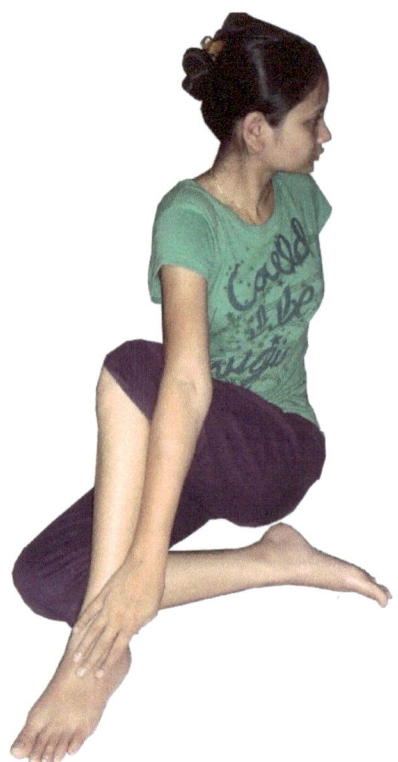

## How to do:

---Sit on the bed with your legs folded

---Now bend your left knee to raise it above the level of bed.

---Place your right hand on your left calf.

---Move your left hand behind your back and look backward as much as you can from over your left shoulder.

--Be in this position for a few minutes.

---Now relax and repeat for the other side of the body.

This is also called "Ardha Matsyendrasana". It's a mild but relaxing pose to start with.

## Spinal Twist

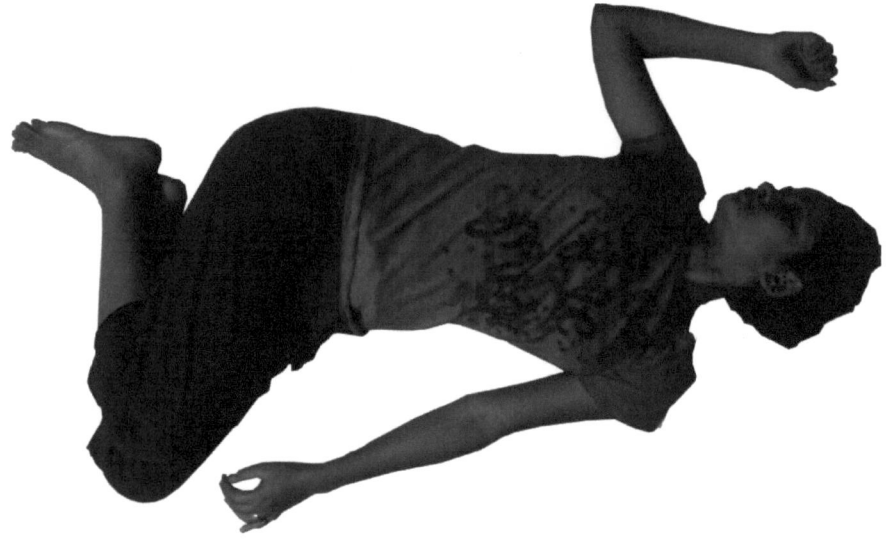

**How to do:**

---Lie down on your back with your arms stretched at a 90 degree angle from your body.(I do not have my hands stretched in this pic)

---Now keep your legs together and bend them on your left.

---Bend your head towards the right as much as you can.

---Be in this position for a few minutes.

---Repeat for the other side.

This posture is also called "Supta Matsyendrasana" and is very very relaxing.
Another one that I used to do unknowingly...

Time for a 'how to **sleep well' tip**...

**Gas** in the stomach can cause a disturbed sleep. Just having fennel seeds after the meals helps in digesting the food faster and bloating doesn't happen.

Another solution is to do this yoga pose after your meals to digest your food easily or if you have gas in your stomach.

## Diamond Pose:

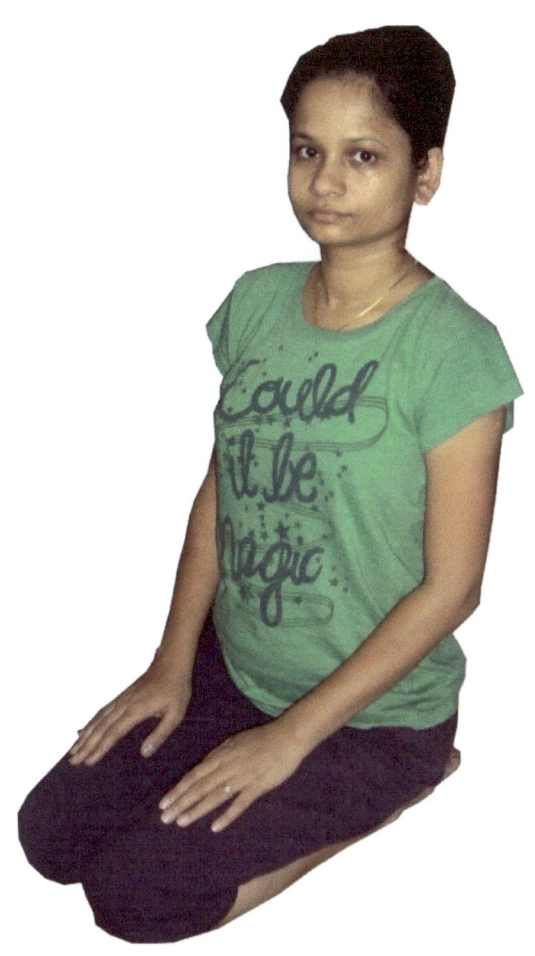

**How to do:**

---Sit down straight.

---Bend your legs backward so that you are sitting on your legs and your feet touch your hips.

---You may keep a pillow between your thighs and calves.

---Relax you arms on your thighs.

---Be in this position for as long as you can. You will feel the difference!!

It's also called "Vajrasana". I, my mom and my sis do it after all our meals.


Now we move to the next posture of yoga for sleep...

# Child's Pose

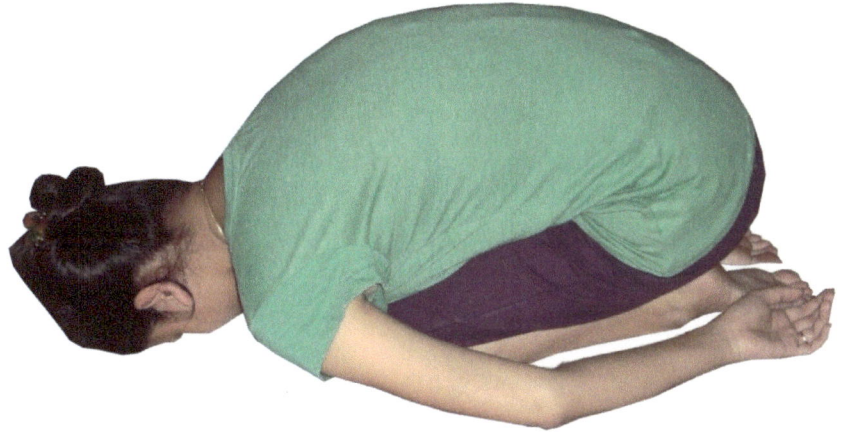

## How to do:

---Sit down and bend your legs backward so that your feet touch your hips. You may keep a pillow between your thighs and calves.

---Now bend forward so that your chest rests on your thighs.

---Bring your hands on the side and relax.

---Now be in this position for a few minutes, breathing normally and then relax.

This posture is also called "Balasana".

I used to do it since childhood not even knowing that it helps me sleep. It's just so relaxing.

Try it for yourself!

# Hand to Foot Pose

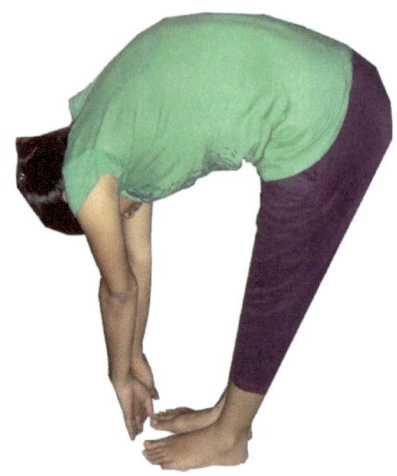

### How to do:

---Stand straight with your hands stretched upwards and legs a bit apart.

---Now exhale and bend forward keeping your knees straight.

---Try touching your feet and have your hands under the feet with your palm facing up. (I can do only this much)

---Now inhale and straighten yourself to initial position.

---Relax and then repeat a few times

This posture is called "Uttanasana"

It may be difficult to touch feet, so one can stretch as much as possible.

# Reclined Tree Pose

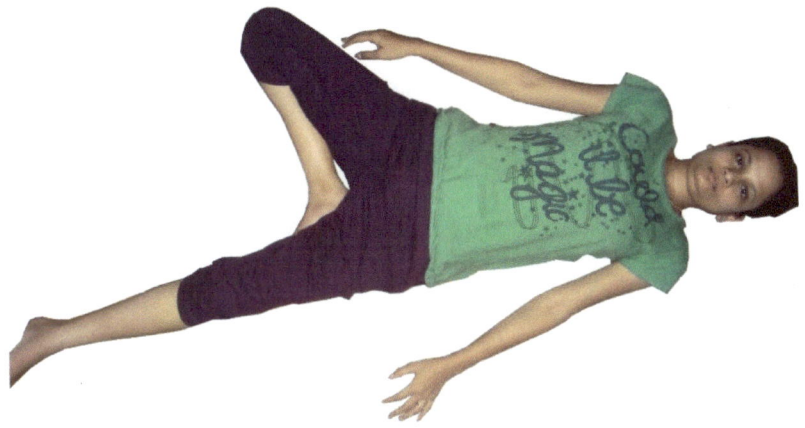

## How to do:

---Lie down on your back with legs straight in front of you.

---Now bend your left foot so that it touches the inner side of the right thigh as shown in the picture.

---Be in this position for a few minutes.

---Now do the same with your right foot.

--Relax and repeat a few times.

This posture is called "Supta Vrksasana".

I used to do this naturally even without realizing that it's a yoga posture! :)

# Cobbler Pose

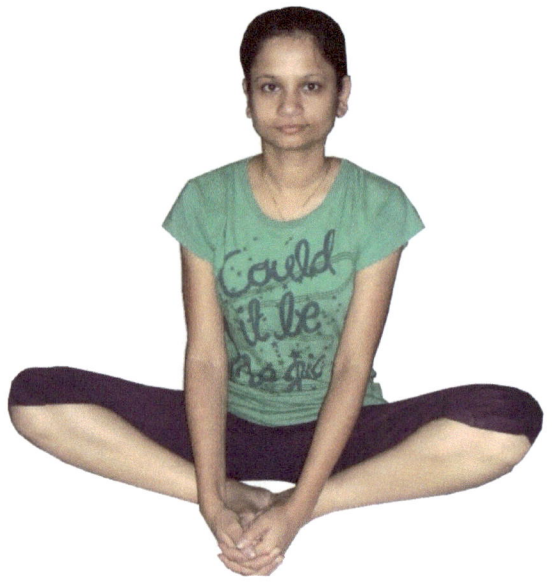

## How to do:

--- Sit straight with your legs stretched in front of you.

---Now bring both the heels closer to the torso with the help of your hands, as shown in the picture. (You may also move your knees up and down while sitting like this)

---Be in this position for a few minutes.

---Relax and repeat.

This is also called "Baddha Konasana". This is an excellent stretching exercise for legs!

An important 'I can't sleep' reason can be...

If men sleep on the side of the bed that's **closer to the door**, they sleep better. And sleeping on the side farther from the door of the room can affect their sleep quality.

That's because men have been protectors, like women have been nurturers. We are wired like that. So, they need to sleep closer to the door to protect from any danger.

# Legs Up

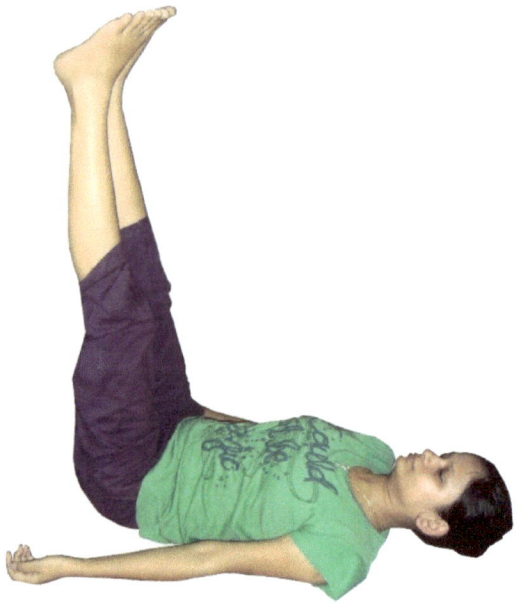

**How to do:**

---Lie down on your back.

---Lift your legs up so that they at 90 degrees with your torso and are straight against a wall. There should not be any space between your hips and the wall.

---Keep your arms a little away from your torso.

---Breathe easy and relax in this position for a few minutes.

---Slowly come to the initial position.

This is also called "Viparita Karani"

# Downward Dog

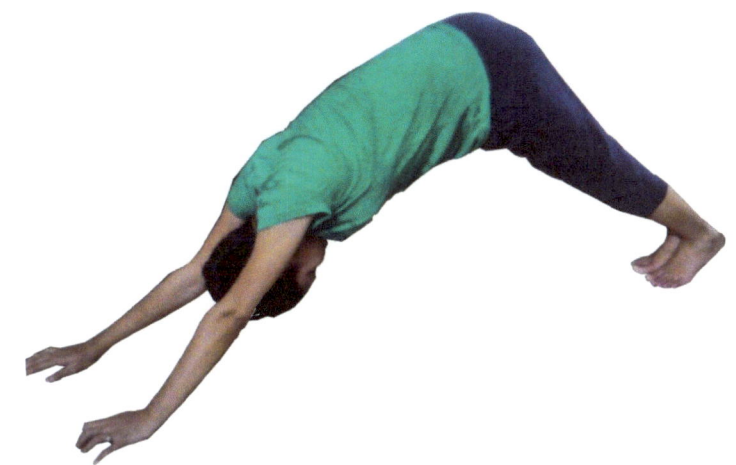

**How to do:**

---Stand straight

---Now bend so that your hands and feet are on the floor

---Make your feet a little apart and your hands too

---Slide the shoulders towards your feet and look in between your feet

---Be in this position for a few minutes and then relax.

This is also called "Adho Mukha Svanasana" and a very good stretching exercise.

## Seated Forward Bend

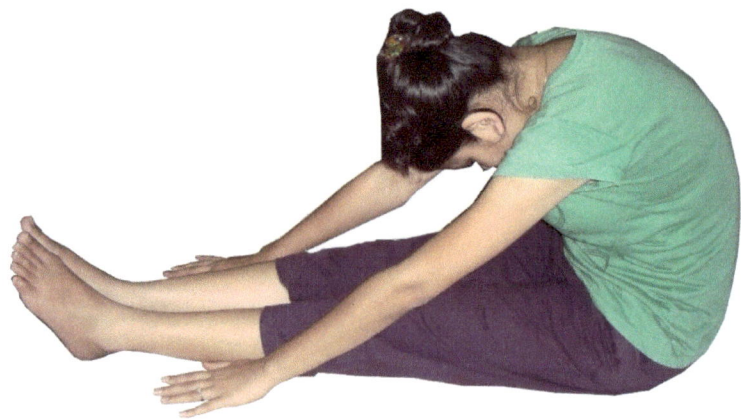

**How to do:**

---Sit on the floor with your legs stretched in front of you.

---Now exhale and bend forward and rest your head on your legs.

---Bring your arms on the side of your body and hold this posture as shown in the picture. If your arms don't reach the feet, stretch them as much as you can. Bending the knees is also an option if necessary.(I can do only this much)

---Be in this position breathing normally for a few minutes and then relax.

This posture is also called "Paschimottanasana"

# Happy Baby Pose

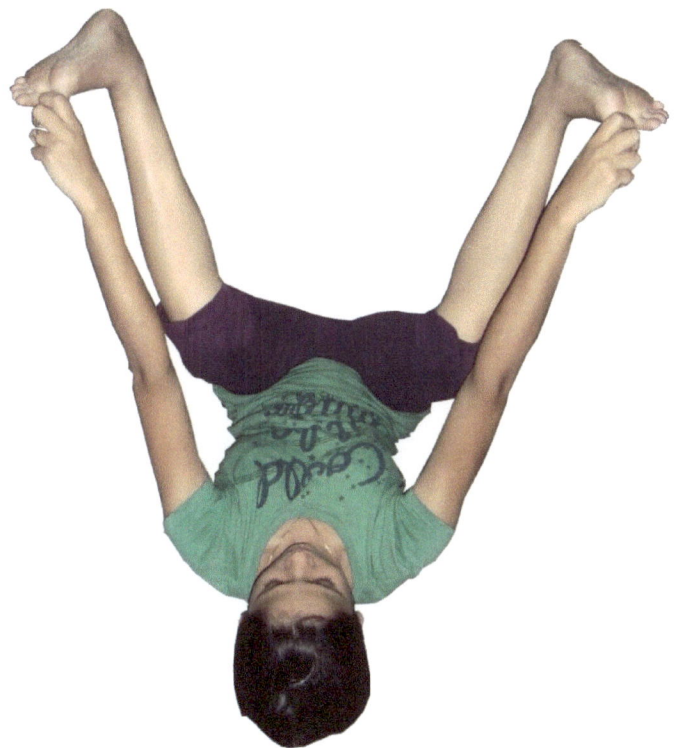

## How to do:

---Lie down on your back

---Now inhale and bend your knees bringing them close to your tummy.

---Now hold your feet with your hands as shown in the picture.

---Be in this position for a few minutes and then exhale and relax

---Repeat a few times.

This posture is also called as "Ananda Balasana", where Ananda means happy and Bala means baby!

# Shoulder Stand

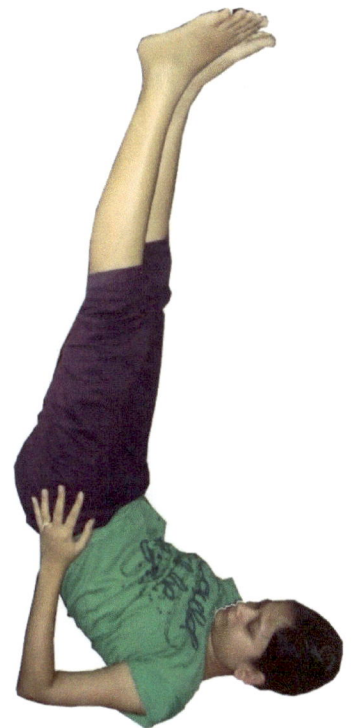

## How to Do:

---Lie down on your back

---Now exhale and slowly lift your body so that only your shoulders are resting on the floor and rest of the body is straight.(I could only do this much)

---Support your body with your hands.

---Be in this position for a few minutes breathing normally.

---Now exhale and relax.

This posture is also called "Sarvangasana". It is considered to be the "Queen of Yoga Aasans".

Though it is a difficult pose, it improves blood circulation and has many more benefits.

That's about the yoga poses for sleep!!! Now let's see how to sleep faster with some...

# Breathing Exercises to Help You Sleep Better

## Single Nostril Breath

How to do:

---Close your left nostril and inhale through the right nostril.

---Now close the right nostril and exhale through the left.

---Repeat for a few minutes - inhaling through right nostril and exhaling through the left.

This one is called *"Suyra Bhedna"* in Hindi language.

Our right nostril represents the heat, or the Sun. *"Surya"* is Sun in Hindi language.

## Another Single Nostril Breath

This is the reverse of the above...

How to do:

---Close your right nostril and inhale through the left nostril.

---Now close the left nostril and exhale through the right.

---Repeat for a few minutes - inhaling through left nostril and exhaling through the right.

This one is called *"Chandra Bhedna"* in Hindi language.

Our left nostril represents the cool, or the Moon. "Chandra" is Moon in Hindi language.

And the last breathing exercise to sleep naturally...

## Alternate Nostril Breathing

How to do:

---Close your left nostril with your thumb and inhale with your right nostril.

---Close your right nostril and exhale with only the left nostril.

---Keep the right nostril closed with your thumb and inhale with the left nostril.

---Close your left nostril and exhale with the right nostril

---Repeat 10 to 15 times

This one is called "*Anulom Vilom*" in Hindi language.

A word of caution...

Please practice these for 2-3 weeks regularly before you expect your sleeping problems getting lesser. They work but you must have patience and consistency!

Now let's see how we can tackle sleep deprivation using...

## Acupressure Techniques

...another natural sleep therapy!

Our bodies have some acupressure points.

Applying little pressure on them for a few minutes helps us relax and handle the sleep problems like insomnia and other sleeping disorders.

Here we go...

Let's see at the back of the head

### Wind Mansion:

It is located in between the two large vertical neck muscles.

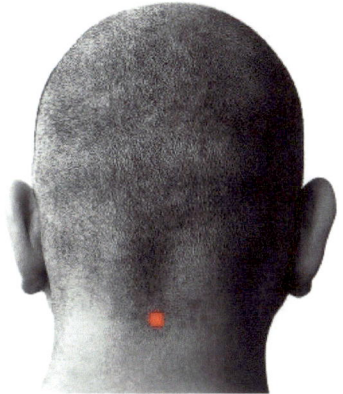

How to find it:

---Bend your head a bit forward. Now try locating two large vertical neck muscles.

---Move your head a bit up and down. You will notice that when you bend the head a bit down a hollow is created between the large neck muscles.

---That's the point under the base of the skull.


Now let's look at the ankle to help you to sleep

**Calm Sleep**

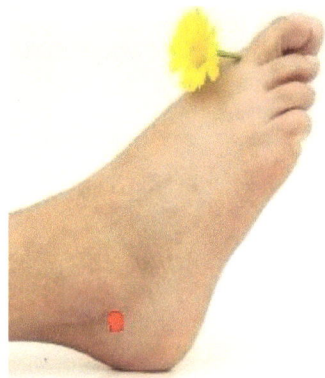

How to find:

---Feel under the outer anklebone. Directly under it there is a little hollow. That's the point.


**Joyful Sleep**

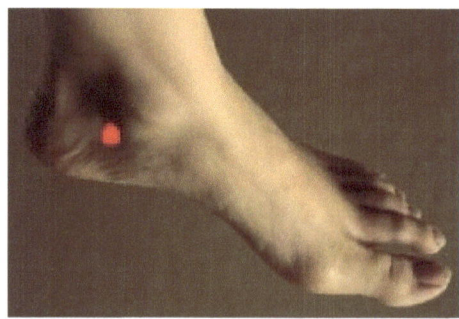

How to find:

---Feel under the inner anklebone. Directly under it there is a little hollow. That's the point.

And on the forehead...

## Third Eye Point

How to find it:

Simple! It's in between the eyes as shown in the picture with the red dot.

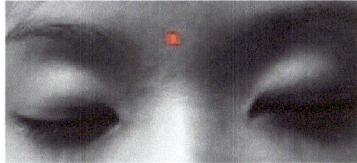

Stay asleep naturally!!! Live well!!!

So, now the question is...

## How much time will it take every day?

You can choose 4-5 of these postures, you are not required to do all of them. Just choose what works best for you.

Do each posture for 1-2 minutes.

So, if you are doing 4-5, it will take a maximum of 10 minutes.

...and 2-3 minutes of breathing exercises and...

... 2 minutes of acupressure.

So, you can sleep easy in **about 15 minutes**.

Won't it be great if 15 minutes can make 'can't sleep at night' a thing of the past? :)

And not just sleep, these yoga poses and breathing techniques will give you a healthier body in the long run!!!

Doesn't it feel so great? :)

...Ok now hunger pangs don't let you fall asleep? Let me tell you some simple and easy...

## Before Bed Snacks

Of course, we don't want to spend time and energy making these...because it's the sleep time!

So, here we go with easy 'sleep like a baby' food...

---Fruits like Banana, raspberries, cherries, avocados and

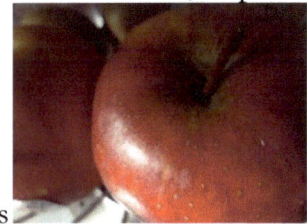

apples

---Oatmeal

---Whole grain cereal with skimmed milk

---Whole grain cracker/toast with a thin layer of peanut butter or almond butter or mozzarella cheese

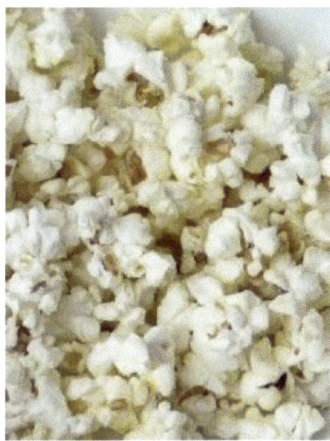

--- ...Popcorn (I simply love them, don't you?)

Some more foods to help you sleep tight...

---Dry fruits like plain almonds 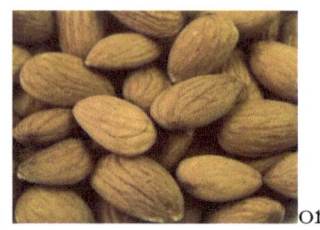 or cashews

---Yogurt

---Cottage cheese

---Chocolate chips

---Granola

And few more so that you don't sleep hungry...

---Hardboiled egg

---Chickpeas

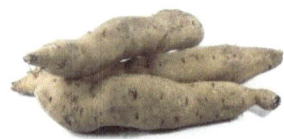

---Sweet potatoes

apart from...

A glass of

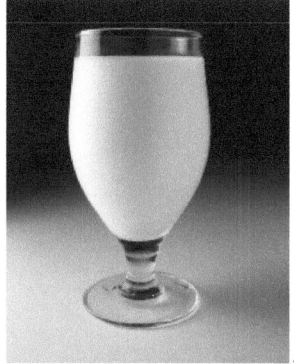...warm milk!! That's a complete sleep diet! Drink it to help you sleep!

You can mix and match them to create interesting foods that help you sleep like shakes, smoothies, sandwiches...

but...

Make sure you have this snack **an hour before you go to sleep**. Don't hit the bed with tummy full or you will be unable to sleep!

Happy Before-bed-Snacking and wish you a sound sleep!! :)

## Natural Insomnia Tips!

So, here we go with our natural sleep remedies...

---Listening to soothing and soft **music** relaxes the mind. So, dim/switch off the lights and put on some soft light soothing sleep music!

---Take **bath** just before going to bed. That relaxes the body. If you are too tired, you may just wash your feet. That also helps in a good night's sleep. I do this all the time, especially in summers!

---Read

...a **book**! ...one which makes you feel sleepy as soon as you pick it up :) Yes, pick one such book, and read it and you will fall asleep!

Make sure it's a physical book, not the one on your laptop or kindle. You can keep that book in your bedside drawer.

---A little

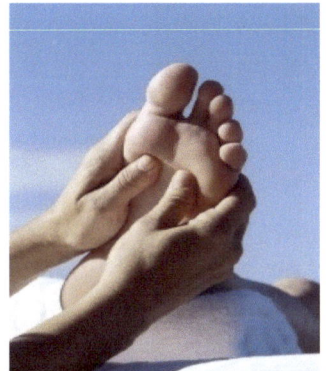
...self **massage** (or massage by someone else) helps a lot in sleeping better! I always had a habit of massaging my feet when I lie down on the bed. That was unconscious but I realize that it helped in me sleeping in no time.

Some more sleep solutions...

---Be in

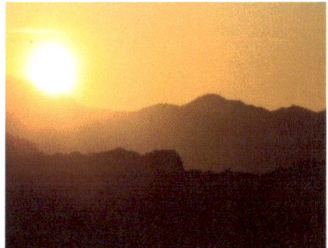
...**sunlight** for an hour or two during the day. Why? Because it helps our bodies produce the sleep hormone, Melatonin, which regulates our sleep.

---Try **aroma therapy**. Just drop 2-3 drops of Chamomile or

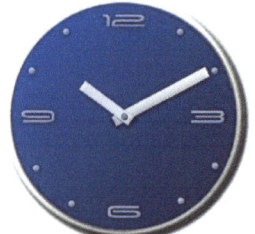...Lavender oil on your pillow - under the pillow cover...Their aroma will help you sleep. You can do it every time you change the cover. Simple and easy! Right?

---Try sleeping and waking up on the

...same time every day. That will suggest to your body that now is the time to sleep and time to wake up. Develop a **sleep schedule** for your body.

---Go to the **washroom** just before going to sleep! That's one of the important sleeping tips.

Some more 'sleep quickly tips'...

---Have some **goals** in life so that you look forward to life when you get up. That gives a feeling of achievement and satisfaction. Important for us to be happy and sleep peacefully!!!

---Little **stretching** of arms and legs helps relax the body. That also helps in sleeping better. But avoid heavy exercising just before going to bed.

---**Meditation** helps in sleep! When I tried it for the first time I slept in less than a minute. What I did was just focus on my breathing for sometime - inhale and exhale...that's it!

A simple sleep meditation technique, isn't it?

What about the bed and the bed room...that's your sleep zone...

---The 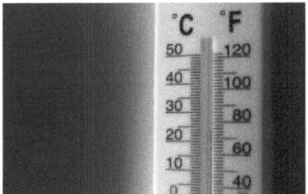...**temperature** of the room must be just right, not hot or cold. Comfortable!

---The

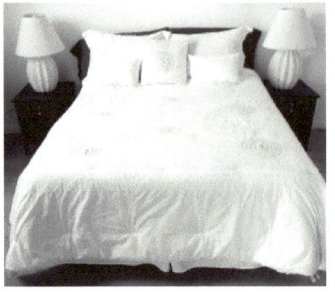 ...**mattress and pillows** should not be too hard or too soft! And too hard or too soft mattress isn't good for spine and neck too!

The ideal way to sleep is without a pillow-yes! Without a pillow! That reduces the chances of neck sprain. I used to have it too frequently, so I'm talking from my personal experience.

---Is your bedroom

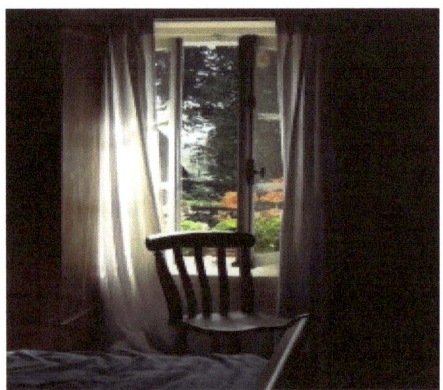 ...well **ventilated**? Make sure it is and there is a window or an inlet for fresh air to come in.

---When you sleep, switch off all the

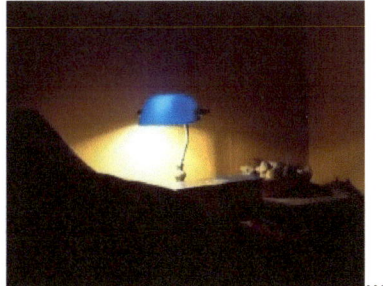... lights. The room should be **dark**, that helps in good sleep! Or you may even use sleep mask on your eyes. Dark room is still preferable.

...and let's talk a bit about **FOOD**...

---Do you eat just before going to bed? Ideally, one must have dinner 2-3 hours before going to bed, so that our body has time to digest the food.

You may have **light bed time snacks** an hour before bed. I share ideas on yum bed time snacks too in this book.

---Heard of have your breakfast like a king and dinner like a beggar? That's true! Eat **light dinner**, heavy dinner will make you feel sleepy but it's not for 6-8 hours of sleep at night.

---Have a glass of

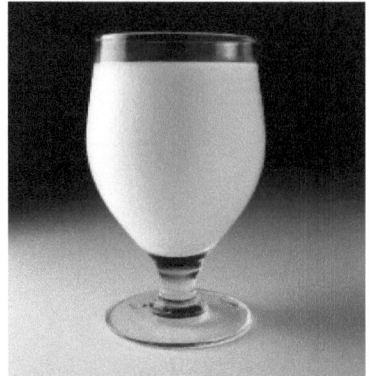

...warm **milk**! It helps in attracting goodnights sleep! Or you may also take a cup of Chamomile or Lavender tea, as it does not have caffeine.

Avoid taking coffee, milk tea (green tea is fine), soft drinks, energy drinks, pain killers, alcohol etc.

---Feel thirsty before bed? That may be because you did not have enough

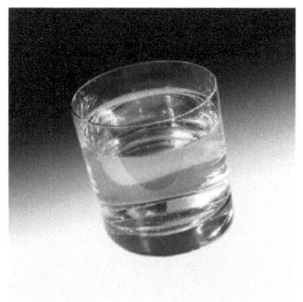

...**water throughout the day**.

So, make sure you have enough water through the day to keep the body well hydrated so that you can avoid liquids before sleep.

...and now is the time for little things to...

# Take Care for a Good Night's Sleep!

---Taking small **naps** during the day reduces the body's need for rest. So avoid that. Let the body get tired during the day so that you feel like sleeping at night.

---Watching

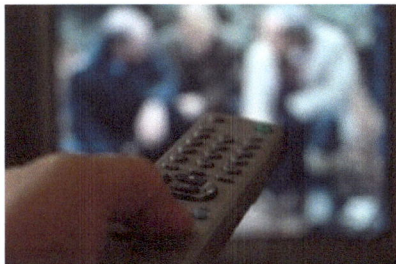
...**TV** especially news or stock market, or anything that disturbs/ stimulates you, hinders with sleep. So, avoid that!

---Try making your

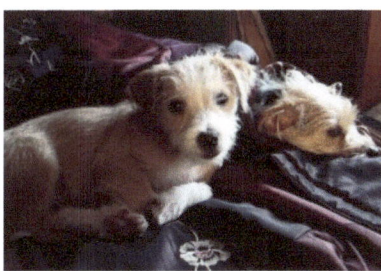
...**pets** sleep in some other room. If you sleep with your pet, it may cause a disturbed sleep.

---We are gadget freaks these days...can't do without

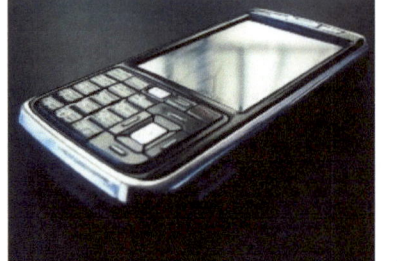

...**cell phones**. Do you know it emits radiations constantly that harm our sleep? So, just keep it at a distance, not just under or near your sleep pillow.

---Do you

...**smoke**? Smokers experience lack of sleep or a more disturbed sleep as compared to non-smokers. So, try that.

...Can I share another trick that has helped me sleep...?

Just lie down to your side and hold **one hand up in the air** straight for a few minutes. You will start feeling sleepy!

---Maintaining personal **hygiene**! That's an important thing in 'how to sleep fast'.

---The **nightwear** has to be comfortable. Yeah for girls I know we want to look smart and comfortable all the time. But comfortable takes precedence here. So, the best clothes for night must be of cotton, soft and comfortable, not body hugging.

---What do you generally **think** about when going to bed? Thinking about your blessings and

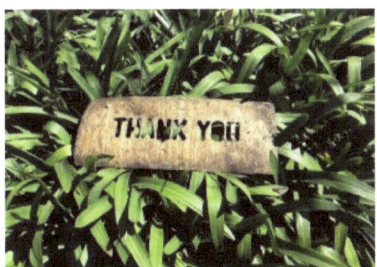

...thanking the almighty for them is one great way to relax and get to sleep...

...and did you know that you will also attract more good things in your life if you sleep your way being grateful for what you have!

---Do you feel

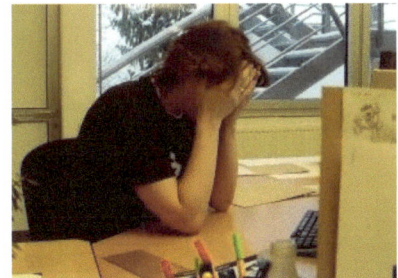

...**stressed**? That will most definitely hinder the sleep. So, try the stress buster ideas that I

share in this book! They worked for me and many people around me, so try them for yourself too!

What about FOOD?

---Do not sleep with a **hungry stomach**! Hunger pangs will keep you awake or wake you up from sleep. So, have some light snack if you wish to. I have a section in this book just for this!

---Foods high in **sugar** content must be avoided before bed.

---Don't drink too much too **liquid before going** to bed. If you do that, then you may have restless sleep because of the need to go to the washroom. So avoid taking in too much liquids just before going to bed.

---Avoid **foods that you are sensitive** to...like foods that may cause acidity, bloating or gas. Have foods that help you sleep, especially 2-3hours before sleep.

...time for a little 'how to get to sleep fast' nugget...

This trick has worked for me sometimes when I can't sleep... (That's very rare though)

Just **blink you eyes slowly** like they are heavy...open them half way and then close...like how it will happen when you are really sleepy. Do that for a few minutes and you will fall asleep! Easy!

And about the bed and bedroom...

---Is your bedroom clean or **cluttered**? A clean bedroom helps in preventing sleep disorders. That's an important part of sleep hygiene!

---What's **under your bed**? Make sure there's nothing or something soft and comfortable like a quilt. If it's some clutter or hard things, you may have trouble sleeping. So, remove it.

---The

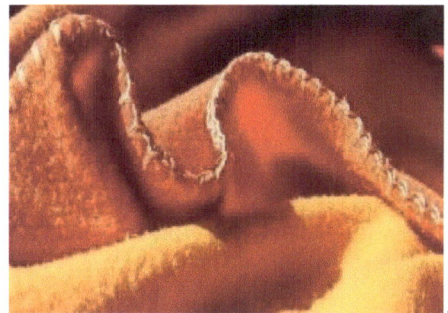
...**blankets** must be of cotton and must be soft so that air can pass through.

---In Feng Shui, it is said that the

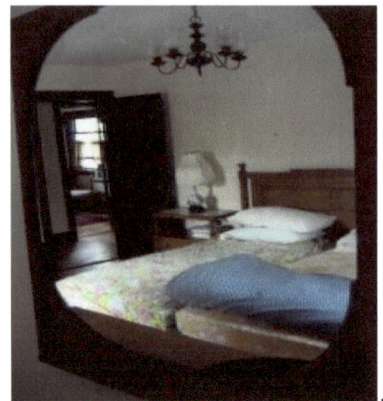...**mirror** in the bedroom should not reflect the bed. One may have disturbed sleep because of that. So, you may move it to some other place or simply cover it with a curtain at night.

---Are there **mosquitoes** in the room where you sleep? Do you use mosquito repellants for it? The best way I suggest is to use a mosquito net. Yes, it requires a little effort before bed but saves you from chemicals and also mosquitoes for sure!

Another thing that I do so that my sleep isn't disturbed...

I have a habit of covering myself with a **blanket**, without that I can't sleep. So, I spread it near me before I go to sleep. Why? Because it wakes me up if I need it and it's kept aside without being spread.

Now let me share with you some practical...

## Stress Buster Ideas

Here are **15 very easily do-able ideas** that will surely help you manage your

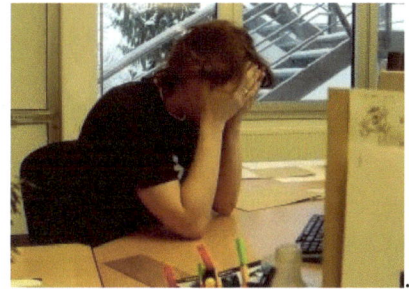...stress or overcoming stress and anxiety from your life!

I have **used them myself** and shared with people. I know they work and that's why I'm sharing them with you!

So, here we go...

--This is a simple one! Just take a

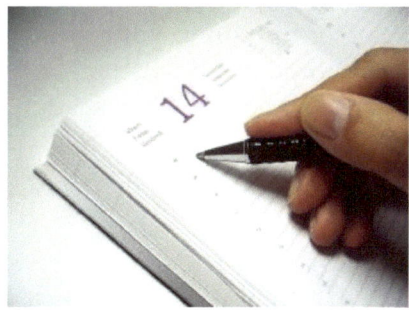...**paper and a pen** (you can also take a diary) and write down whatever comes to your mind...it can be anything at all, just let it out.

When we keep on thinking about a situation, it just keeps us stressed...when we take it out on the paper, it stops revolving in our head and we feel relaxed. Simple! Isn't it?

I told this to 2 of my friends and the very next day they called to thank me because they slept like babies after so long :) ...and I have been using it since always!

---**Talk**!

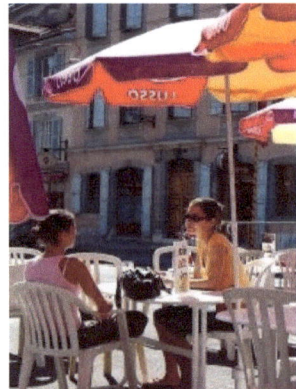...Yes, just talk to the person because of whom you are feeling stressed.

Talking will help **releasing what's going on in your mind** and may be they have a different viewpoint for whatever they did/said, listen to their side of the story as well while sharing yours.

Don't get into a blame game though!

I have tried this so many times. Particularly when my husband says something, I interpret it my way and then I start building around that in my mind and start feeling stressed. The moment I talk to him how I am feeling, I realize he never meant it the way I took it or has a reason for it. So, talking helps a long way!

### ---**Gratitude**-

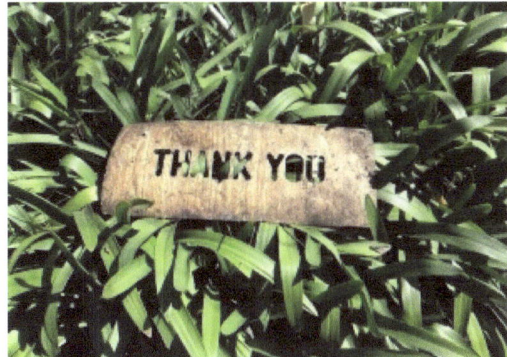

...This one is huge!

Look around yourself - You are bound to have people/things/situations that you are thankful for. One is that you are alive and have eyes to read this book. Many people don't have even that!

So, count your blessings and relax. This will help you feel less stressed and sleep happier!

---Many a times, we think of the **worst situations** and get stressed unnecessarily. Such situations don't even happen!

Let me share an example with you. In my office, once my manager took some action and I felt that I will be out of job for no fault of mine. And I was terribly stressed out for 2 days.

Then I just thought let me speak to my manager. And she said she had to take that action but that will not have any impact further.

Phew! **What stressed me, never happened**! Do you see the point? :)

A few more ideas for stress relief...

---Are you the kind of person who has **too many things** on her/his plate and feel stressed because of that? Let me share a simple solution with you that has worked wonders for me...

Just make a

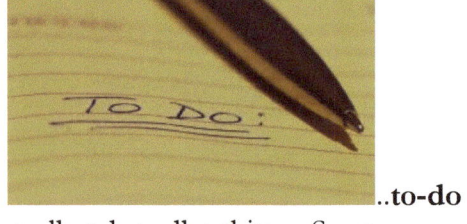 **..to-do list** with all the big and small and smaller things. So, now you won't forget anything. Now, see what's most important and start doing them and ticking them priority-wise.

Listing everything down relaxes to the extent we can't even imagine! Try it sometime!

---This is something that I love! No matter what happens, just think **will it matter** in the long run, say 5 years from now? Mostly the answer will be "No"! So, when it doesn't matter in the long run, let it be, be easy!

---**Sleep over it** -

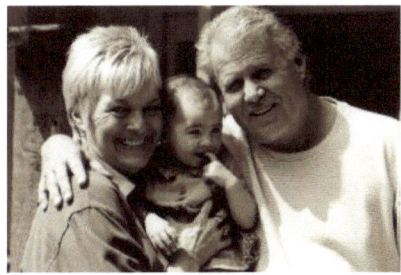

...The issue will seem smaller when you get up the next morning! There are bad days when we or the other person overreacts. So, sleep over it and it will be fine.

--- Deep **breathing** helps in relaxing our body. In daily life we don't breathe deep as much as we should. So, try this for a few minutes.

And more to living stress free life...

---Spend time with **family** -

...little kids, elders (grandparents) and your pets. They give unconditional love always! And kids and elderly people also have interesting stories to tell from their life ;)

---Do **something that you love to do** - Like playing some musical instrument, or singing, dancing, cooking, gardening, some sport, swimming or may be photography...something that you enjoy!

---Spend time with

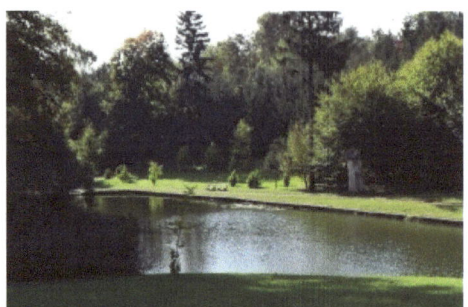

...**nature** - go for a walk barefoot or trekking or on a beach to watch sunset. Isn't that so relaxing?

---Have a glass of

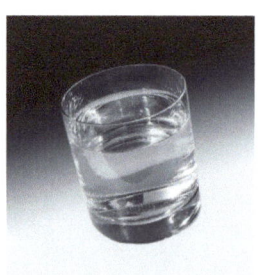

...**water**! ...and cool down! :)

Apart from these, to get rid of stressful life...

--- Go for a **drive**! Not on roads with traffic of course!

---Take a week **long break** and go spend some leisure time. You deserve it!

---Go to a

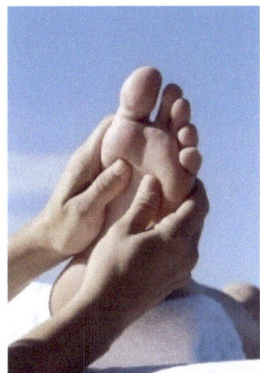

...**spa** and get a full body massage! Wow! It's always so relaxing! Try that one?

# About the Author

Hi there!

I'm Suchi from India.

I see so many people who don't get sound sleep or no sleep at all. That included my husband Saket too.

I get scared by the very thought of lying on the bed in dark wide awake and waiting for sleep and it feels like a never-ending wait...checking the time again and again and realizing only a few minutes passed by...

Phew! It just doesn't feel right or good! What if I was in that situation...that thought scares me so much...and I can understand how restless and frustrating it would feel.

People around me say I'm **blessed** to have baby sleep every night and they would wish the same for themselves.

So, I thought why not share with YOU what I do (naturally, it's been my habit always- unconsciously) to be blessed with a goodnight's sleep.

That's where this 'how to sleep better' guide was born!

I'm a die-hard fan of **natural remedies**. So, in this book I share with you some natural ways to get a good sound sleep! Best Yoga Poses for Sleep and other sleep techniques like breathing, acupressure and many many tips.

### No sleeping tablets, no doctors!

So, here's the book for you - a compilation of natural 'how to sleep well' aids which can be done at home without the need to spend money.

I truly hope you also find it helpful on 'no sleep' nights. **Anyone can do it**…just a little bit of 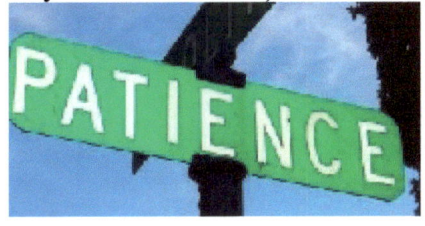 is required!

Would you like to share your "From Sleep Deprivation to Sleep Tight" experiences with me? Please drop a line at replytosuchi at yahoo dot com. I would love to hear from you!

All the very best for your journey towards deep sleep! :)

Good Night, Sleep tight!!!

Suchi Gupta

## Other books by the same author

"8 Effective Yoga Postures to Lose Belly Fat "
Available at  http://amzn.com/B007VJ7K24

# Attributions

The pictures that I have used in this "how to go to sleep fast" book have been taken from http://www.sxc.hu. They have been clicked by:

Sam Hatch - The Baby Sleeping Picture

Foxumon - The money picture

Ivan Prole – The time picture

Tom Pickering - The patience picture

Tonypowell - The apples picture

Brian Lary - The almonds Picture

Shannah Pace - The popcorn Picture

Vangelis Thomaidis - Sweetpotato Picture

Bev Lloyd-Roberts - The pets Picture

Dcarson924 - The foot-massage Picture

Richard Dudley - The glass-of-water picture

Janet Burgess - The Talk-it-out picture

Lavinia Marin - The pen-n-paper picture

Kimberly Appelcline - The Gratitude picture

Masha_L - The nature picture

Jocilyn Pope - The sleep-over-it picture

Stacie Andrea - The grandparents picture

barun patro - The cellphone picture

Bartek Ambrozik - The time picture

Mateusz Stachowski - The to-do-list picture

Davor Fanton - The Temperature Picture

Pascal THAUVIN - The blanket picture

Ddrccl - The Matress-n-Pillow picture

Mi-sio - The cigarette picture

Jamie Hansen - The compass picture

Getupgirl - The mirror-bed picture

Pontus Edenberg - The dark room picture

Pete 'Langy' Langshaw - The Lavendar picture

Nicci Hampton - The ventilation picture

Uros Kotnik - The milk glass picture

Sias van Schalkwyk- The book picture

Sem rox - The TV picture

Thomas van den Berg - The sunrise picture

Carl dwyer - The stress picture

SandyYin - Eyes closed Picture

Cecilia picco - Bald-head picture

Leagun - The foot picture

Ramzi hashisho_foot picture

Thanks to all these wonderful photographers for letting me utilize their pictures in this 'sleep help' book.